PSORIASIS AND THE TRUTH

The Secret to Overcoming Psoriasis

By J. Thegg

Health Information Specialist

RHIT, CPC, CCS

INTRODUCTION

We want to thank you for purchasing this book, "Psoriasis: The Truth". This book contains proven steps and strategies on how to eliminate Psoriasis from your life. With two meals you can change your well-being for the better. In this book you will find out the facts about psoriasis from an experienced researcher and a previous psoriasis sufferer.

Thanks again for purchasing this book, we hope you enjoy it!

FOR A FREE LIST OF 100 MEDICINAL HERBS TO GROW EASILY AND QUICKLY TO:

1. USE IN TEA OR COOKING

2. GROW IN A SMALL GARDEN

3. HERBS FOR ANY AILMENT

Visit: NurseOasis.com and scroll to bottom or go to: **https://tinyurl.com/y96g9ocb**

Printed in the United States of America

First Printing, 2016

First Edition

DEDICATION

I want to thank my little dog, Gracie, who died June 30th at 9:20 am, 2016 for showing me love and allowing me to feel love for once in my life. I wrote this book after her passing to resolve my heart and let readers know that if you feel good within your body, anything is possible. I miss my little love so much and it hurts every day, but I try to keep going, one step at a time. What was left after this heart wrenching tragedy is my health and without that, well, I would have probably joined her. Here is my true story how I cured psoriasis with my Biotechnology background to come up with 2 simple meals that changed my life.

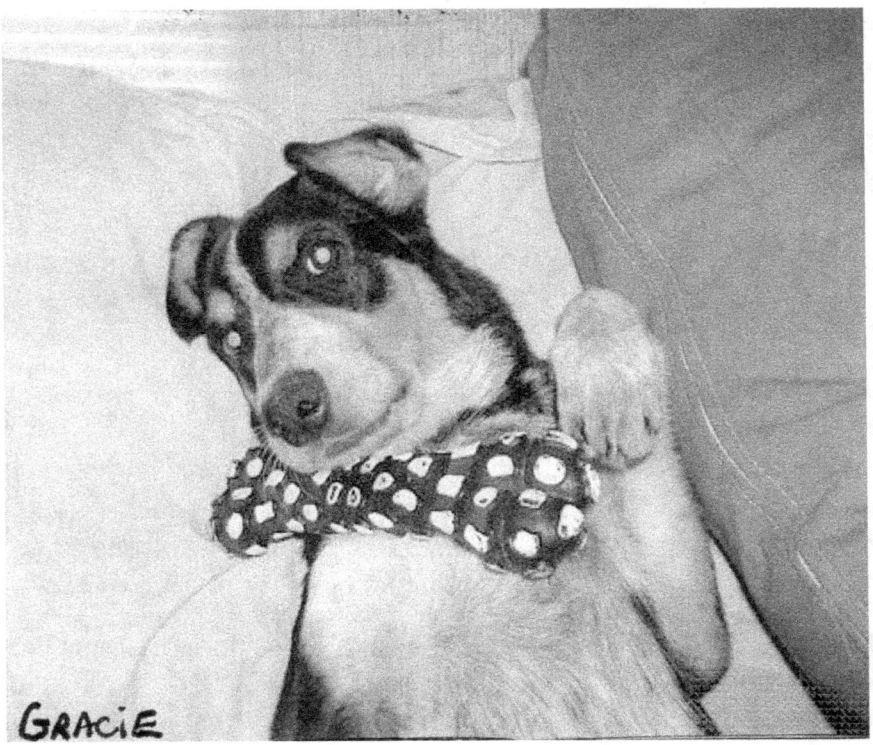

GRACIE

PREFACE

After so many Doctor visits my psoriasis had progressed to my face, and doctors said it usually never goes to the face. It did on me. Psoriasis took over my life completely. I realized and remembered I took Biotechnology classes. I did research on many things, why not this. That is when I said no more. Psoriasis took 30+ years of my life. I finally had the courage to believe in myself in order to cure myself and in this book, you will read what I found out. God Bless you.

By Understanding the reason skin conditions occur you can find out how to super boost your strength, and have the ability to handle stress, while gaining incredible information to keep with you for the rest of your life. You can leave Psoriasis behind knowing about simple combined spices (https://nurseoasis.com/spices-to-your-liking) and 2 simple meals. Please visit our website for the freshest spices. Goodbye Psoriasis, Hello to the Beautiful You!

Is psoriasis really an autoimmune disease? Or is it a money-making disease? In the dictionary, autoimmune disease listed description as follows:

Immune system **disorders** cause abnormally low activity or over activity of the **immune** system. In cases of immune system over activity, the body attacks and damages its own tissues (**autoimmune diseases**).
Immune deficiency **diseases** decrease the body's ability to fight invaders, causing vulnerability to infections' 7, 2016

Ok, I'll go for that. However, if it is an autoimmune disease, why does it only attack certain members of a family? Why is the body attacking itself? The answer is simple.

Let me start from the beginning. You don't have to have a bad childhood to get psoriasis. People that have psoriasis are usually hard-working and dedicated individuals with probably more character than the people directly surrounding them. Why? Because people with psoriasis think more than most people. They worry about the future and their actions that will shape the future. People with psoriasis worry about preventing things from not going their way. People with psoriasis have a conscious and want to do the best they can. They took their stress to the next level and did not stop to relax. While others relax, the psoriasis sufferer keeps going and going, only to get their pH out of balance.

People that stress out, do not eat right, and ignore pain within their bodies that do not develop psoriasis, will more than likely get disease later on in life as they get older.

Eating fast food does not help the situation. Ever notice when you are stressed out and very busy, we tend to stop by fast food places to hurry up and eat to get to the next chore we need to do before the day is over? You are what you eat; the phrase is true even today.

Don't fret, you don't have to give up fast food. In fact, all you have to do is eat the right meal to help your body get back to a normal pH balance and stay there for a longer period. The body will begin to train itself to remain in pH balance. Disease cannot live in our bodies with a normal pH balance. Once your body is out of balance for a long period and has developed psoriasis, it is hard to get it back. You have to work twice as hard and long to reach a complete balance that will last long term. In this book is a quick and 100% natural way to achieve this goal.

With instruction, you can eat one meal and see long term results. Let us show you how to make psoriasis a bad memory. Keep reading.

TABLE OF CONTENTS

CHAPTER 1: A MEMORABLE CHILDHOOD

HOW OUR CHILDHOOD EXPERIENCES AFFECT OUR SKIN

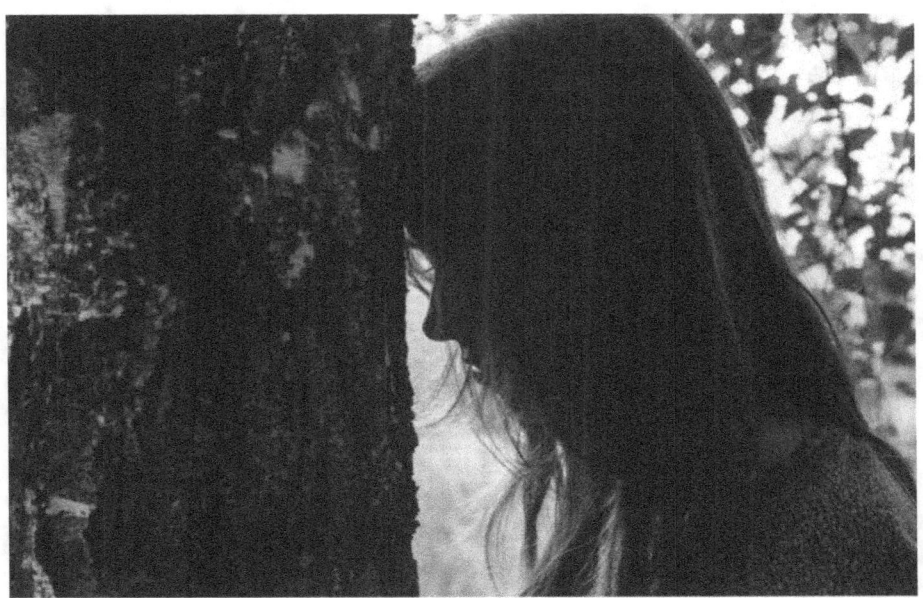

Experiences in our childhood are very important. If you have abuse anywhere in your family, it can affect your entire life. Negative or positive, we do not leave our childhood memories in the past; it comes with us as adults. Most of the time, our character and personality are shaped or hindered by our childhood.

We have to learn to distinguish in which manner experiences affect our lives. First, it is important to accept the good experiences, and try to accept the ones that are not good. There are experiences that change our lives in a critical way. In most cases, we remember experiences that are sad and traumatic. Sadness may promote all kinds of fears that we have to learn to beat. We have to learn to accept every bad situation that resulted in a negative experience. That is very difficult to do, especially for a child.

Two different people may share the same experience but interpret them differently. Depending on their personality and character, people react differently to different situations. Some people can simply brush off negativity, while others take it more seriously. All we can do is learn from all the experiences we encounter and do the best we can to be happy. Not an easy task for anyone.

Blaming our childhood usually can get us off the hook. But today we have to stand on our own, be sincere and look at our faults while trying to change them for the better. It is important not to look too much at our faults and how they occurred but try to calm the mind and realize it's over. We must be truthful with ourselves and everyone around us. Just have the intention and ask for help if you can. Do not look at the cause of your character because it's the past, but rather try to change negative thinking to better your life and others around you. All we need is to have the motive and inclination to do it.

It is important to mention again that we should not blame our experiences but try to learn from them. Because we now know every experience will affect us, either negative or positive, it is important to take the good with the bad. Of course, it's easier said than done for everyone. No one is immune to this difficulty.

Reminisce of the days of being a child. What comes to mind? Frolicking through the forest, connected to nature? Feeling free and innocent? Basically, what society views childhood to be? The fact is some children go through a living hell. Many children have less than perfect childhoods, dealing with abuse or with an abused parent, such as myself. It is written that for every ten seconds that go by, a child is abused. Loss of self-esteem, acting out negatively, and lack of confidence all stem from our parents if they are abusers. It's a good thing we can write about it and express our emotions into words.

Neglect is the most common abuse. The psychological (mental and emotional) state of being neglected includes lack of support and love, especially when you love your parents and they don't really show you love back. We are simply too young and vulnerable to know the difference at the time it is happening. Parents that never express some type of support to their children end up molding their children to be what they are, positive or negative. Unfortunately, society does not care either. We must search for answers; seek and hopefully we will find. This is exactly what happened to me. Horrible neglect was my payment in life. The type of neglect you do not even know is happening. In child neglect, you are simply too young to know what neglect is until it's too late and you are much older.

My father was a booze-drinking-could-not-care-less type of person that worked every day and only thought about himself most of the time. My father was a wife abuser. My mother was a neurotic, whining, self-proclaimed victim who maybe would have done more with her life if she had the internet back in the 70's. Who really knows what excuse she would have come up with for not learning and getting out of such an abusive marriage? She suppressed her abuse and emotions with valium, which was accepted and normal back then.

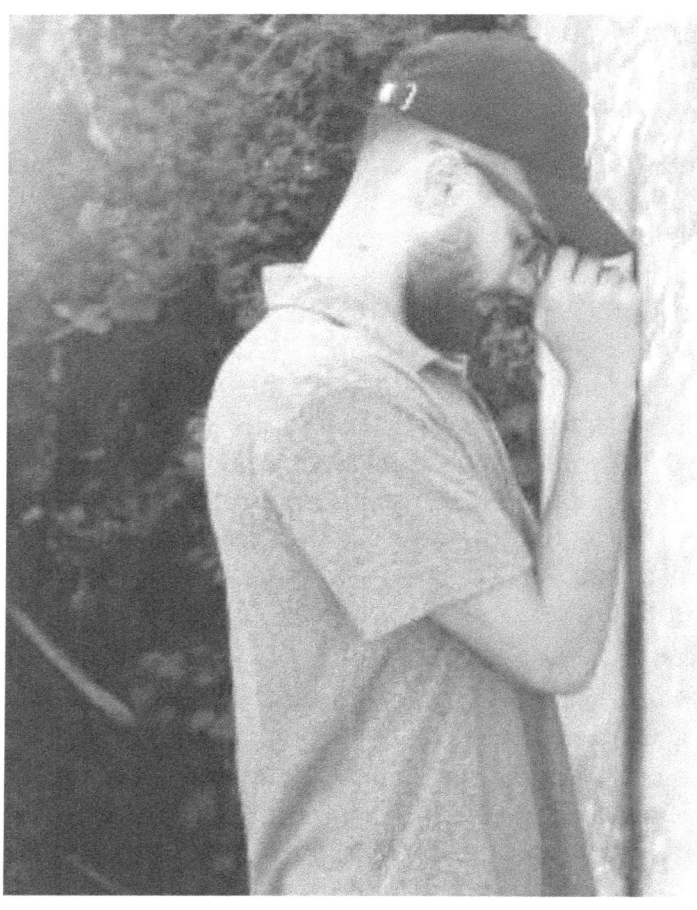

Guilty as charged. No personal relationship existed between husband and wife or parents and children at all. After the OJ Simpson trial, now domestic abuse is more recognized and dealt with much more rapidly.

What I found out next shocked me. All that sadness built up and built up into tension, frustration, and ultimately released through my skin. I had horrible chronic psoriasis most of my childhood and teen years. Read on to find out the how and why built up tension will lead to disease or better yet, skin inflammation. Skin Inflammation is a sign that signifies you are on "overload" and a great indicator to future disease. It's a sign from the body to yours truly, saying, "Hey, I love you, but we must calm down."

CHAPTER 2: STRESS AND PSORIASIS

THE TRUTH ABOUT PSORIASIS

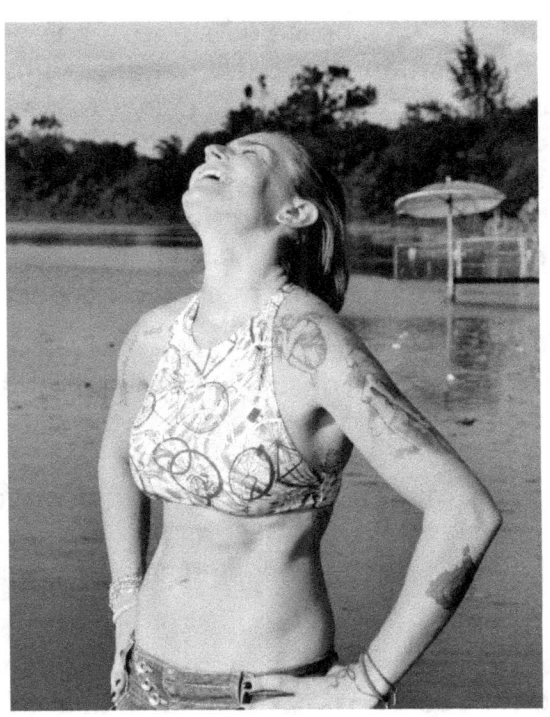

The body follows the mind. Mental distress can affect human function better known as physiology. Elevated adrenaline and cortisol that are released during stress will lead to hormonal imbalance and unresolved inflammation. Anger, fear, and anxiety are typically stored and expressed in the gut.

"I'm so stressed out!" You have probably said those words many times, but it is important to realize what that exactly means. When we hear the word "stress", you picture someone at their end of patience and pulling their hair out. Stress is a combination of responses within the body. There are three different categories of stress. The first is acute stress, the second is chronic stress, and the third is psychological stress. What doctors refuse to let their patients know is that stress must "build up" to become psoriasis. It may take months or years. Daily stress builds and builds and builds and finally it must go somewhere. The result is illness or skin inflammation.

We are referring to the complicated surge of chemicals that rush through the body when we get frustrated, angry, helpless, lonely, or depressed. We are focusing on things like our children, crisis resolutions, and taking instant action to resolve things. Acute stress happens when our bodies are focused on something immediate concerning the resolution of a crises situation. Humankind would not live long if it was not for instant action our bodies take in a fight or flight response. Acute stress can be helpful and can save lives.

The two factors present in stress are internal and external. Stressors are present in external stress, which are situations or circumstances that cause stress as an external stimulus. These external stressors may be linked to too much work, too little money, too many creditors, the arrival of a baby, or the excitement of a new job. External stresses have a heavy impact on the handicapped.

A person that is handicapped is more vulnerable to stress and tension for obvious reasons. Feeling vulnerable to external and environmental difficulties is harder for a handicapped person; therefore, psoriasis can develop very quickly. The buildup of medications taken daily increase fatigue and decreases the mind's ability to cope with daily activities. One must detox and detox safely, not quickly. It took a long time for medications to build up and can be eliminated quickly if you know what to do. We will show you in this reading.

Stress becomes dangerous to humans when it enters the category of internal stress or chronic stress. There are an infinite number of situations that can cause chronic stress, such as relationships or family problems, high expectations on the job, not enough rest, and many other circumstances. Usually, people do not know what is happening to them when chronic stress surfaces. The human brain is programmed to direct your body on how to react to all types of stress, but it cannot differentiate between whether the stress is something to run from or sit still for. Chronic stress affects many organs in the body negatively. Along with the brain, heart, lungs, and digestive system, whether it's good or bad, external or internal, it's all the same stress and it's building on top of itself within the body without our knowledge.

Stress can lead to periodontal disease. Stress can cause hormonal changes and psychological (mental and emotional) stress plays a big role in periodontal disease. In 1960, research discovered that hormonal imbalance, nutritional imbalance, and diabetes; all can cause periodontal disease. The study also shows that stress has everything to do with it. Stress allows the release of adrenaline, heart rate increase, increased respiration, and other physiological (chemical) signals. It is important to know that when stress or tension is prolonged for long periods of time, it will lead to periodontal disease and other diseases. Gum disease is known as "opportunistic infections" that can develop under physiological (chemical) conditions known as stress. Therefore, the role of stress in periodontal illness has been proved and warrants attention (Wrigleyville).

Periodontal disease has microorganisms that lead to inflammation reflex. Gingivitis is periodontal disease, which begins with inflamed gums. Bacteria will cause periodontal disease, but stress is the forefront which starts the disease developing. Stress also prevents the healing of periodontal wounds.

There are many situations that can cause stress and there are two main sections. Physical Stressors are factors that produce stress through physical means. This can mean when a person is physically hot, cold, hungry, or in pain due to an infection.

Psychological Stressors are everyday situations not caused by physical means. Examples of this are loss of job, death of a family member, separation from a loved one, or financial hardship.

Stress itself is defined by both psychological and physiological factors. Psychological means dealing with the mental or emotional state of a person. Physiological deals with the body and its organs. Psychological stress is a result of many factors and should be dealt with very carefully. Stress can be defined as a set of interactions between the person and the environment that result in an unpleasant emotional state, such as anxiety, tension, guilt, or shame. Another way of putting it; there are some things that put certain demands on us. Many studies have concluded that the effects on our physical health from stress can be extremely detrimental. These adverse physical effects include heart disease and formations of cancer. There are numerous elements that trigger the effects of psychological stress. Having too many credit card payments, relationship or employment problems, can all lead to stress out of our control. The effects of stress should not be limited to bad emotional states, but this type is the most damaging to our bodies.

Frustration is one of the elements that will start stress. Frustration is one of the most constant sources of stress. Many different situations will provoke frustration. Frustration can occur when something is blocking fulfillment of our needs or goals. All of the everyday things that frustrate us include sense of failure, death, loneliness, inadequacies, bad relationships, and waiting in lines of traffic. Self-demeaning thoughts can be a way we sabotage ourselves which may block getting our needs met. Sometimes we convince ourselves that we are not able to reach our goals, or someone could not possibly love us, and we can create a self-fulfilling prophecy. We do have the ability to change negative thinking, but it seems easier said than done. Positive or negative life changes can lead to stress in different ways. Today, many people fall into an everyday routine and fear change to that routine. For people uncomfortable with change, it can be stressful and sometimes traumatic. I think most people will agree that any change causes stress. Starting a new car is stressful. Stress causes and factors have been studied by many people. Stress is a very vague condition to recognize and many scholars have studied it and come up with different categories to help classify what type of stress is being suffered. Stress may be chronic, for example, poverty or other difficult living conditions that are ongoing in one's life. Stress can also be transitory, an act such as a noise that bothers a person. Lastly, stress depends on the individual. Different types of stress can cause different reactions in different people. The fact is that certain situations may cause people to feel negative and react in a negative manner if they feel external or internal pressure. Many instances of tension, mental or physical, have something to do with people dealing with other people which can be the majority of the pressure.

Stress is normal in life. No one is immune to stress and what is causes. The way we handle stress is so important especially today with so much going on. Some ignore their problems while others face them head on. Stress and frustration can either cause harm or make you who you are. We all have different stressors that cause stress. At some point, stress will become chronic if not dealt with. Being late or driving too fast can cause a person to be rude while driving. Parents who ignore their children that are too loud and need discipline or attention can cause stress. Having many duties or accountabilities during each day, an ill parent or child, medical emergency, stolen property or vehicle, bankruptcy or unemployment, and being handicapped are only a few reasons we become extremely unbalanced. This is the cause of chronic tension within the body that builds up and up and up. This building up and up of disease-causing hormones and proteins will continue until we find a way to start over. Here is where our Awesome Kernel Mix (http://amzn.to/2DTKNdw) comes in to the rescue! Eating our delicious 9-lentil mix meal allows the body to delete, reset, and start over; this is very important for optimal health.

In today's fast pace environment, happiness is signified by materialistic means and pursuing them takes plenty of mental and physical energy as well as dealing with financial burdens. This causes stress in life whether we are aware of it or not. This type of stress results in a continuous state of tension.

This happened to me and resulted in my chronic psoriasis. I had no idea how much stress I was under growing up. Nobody cared enough to show me the way in life, and I was destined for buildup of disease. Good for you, I am writing this book to let you know what I found out, what I realized, and how I found the best solution for get rid of psoriasis. My background in Biotechnology research came in very handy when I started researching why psoriasis happens in the first place.

CHAPTER 3: WHY DETOX IS SO IMPORTANT

HOW YOUR BODY IS UNDER CONSTANT ATTACK

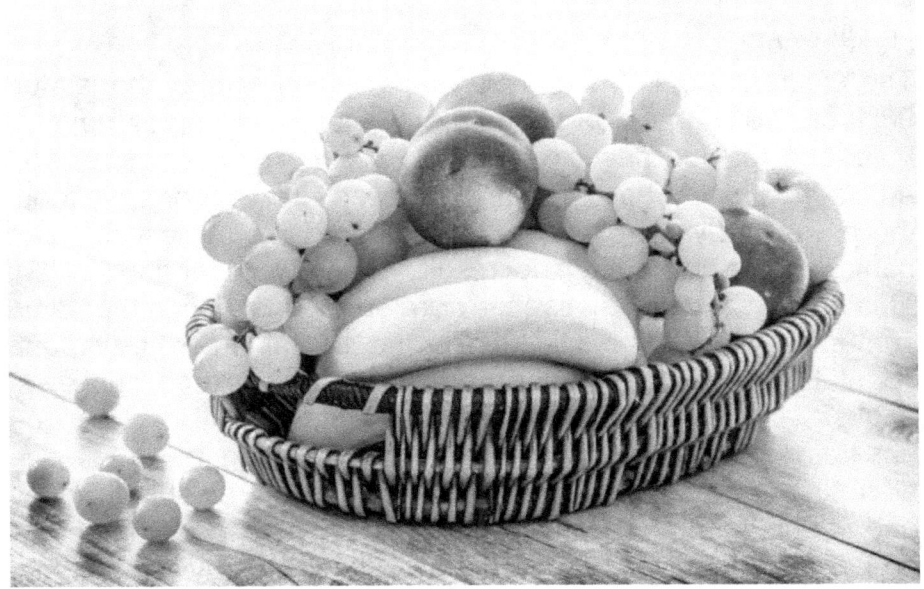

Let's begin with pesticides. Pesticide is a known poison, designed to kill pests and insects. Pesticides contain the chemical organophosphate, which is the main ingredient in nerve gas. The same nerve gas used in war battles (Biddle). Pesticides have been especially designed to kill insects and damage their nervous systems. They work by altering an enzyme in the insect that has to do with nerve function. However, the same result can occur in humans when eating foods or vegetables that contain residual pesticide amounts.

Large companies that supply food to the population all use pesticides to kill insects because it increases the yield of their crops. This means more profitability for their business. However, they do not concern themselves with what they are doing to our families. We end up eating nerve poison. Remember, this pesticide was created to stay on top of crops or go inside the crop and withstand rain and deterioration. This is not good, not good at all for us. When this pesticide is put on crops, it is designed to not wash off with the rain, and that is what we digest in our bodies every day. The pesticide is a type of wax put on the crops. We end up eating it.

Need proof?
The Environmental Working Group published a study that stated 98% of strawberries, peaches, nectarines, and apples have at least one residue pesticide left when at the grocery store. The article mentioned, however, that when children ate organic food, the pesticides were eliminated. Small amounts of pesticide can damage a young child and result in ADHD or worse (EWG). This article says the levels today are safe but states in the same sentence that wax pesticide residue contained in fruits and vegetables today can cause harm to young children and even adults. This means the exposure to these pesticides can be unsafe and they are just reporting it, not stopping it. Can we use all-natural pesticides? The large companies are all about money and time is money. It is not known exactly why food companies do not take a more natural approach, though many are starting, but limited to small farms.

Since fruits and vegetables may contain 146 different types of pesticides, the concern is the nerve gas contained in these dangerous insect-killing products that have negative effects on children with vulnerable brain function. Long-term use can result in long-term damage to the brain or nervous system. It is mentioned that pesticides in foods rarely cause visible illness but also state that young children with developing nervous systems can be negatively affected (EWG).

Pesticides do not just enter the body by food. Between 1992 and 2001, the US Geological Survey found that pesticides pollute every stream that was sampled, and more than 90% of all wells. Pesticide residues were also found in rain and groundwater (US Geo). This means that every time we drink water, we are probably drinking nerve poison too! The end result is chronic toxicity, which may lead to delayed or altered memory, chronic depression, irritability, confusion, headaches, insomnia, nightmares, nausea, disorientation of concentration, exhaustion, fatigue, and an overall feeling of weakness. For children, ingesting pesticide residues may result in delayed learning abilities, lack of physical coordination, behavioral and developmental problems, including ADHD. All facts for each pesticide are documented within Extoxnet's "Pesticide Information Profiles" report (Extoxnet).

In 2011, the Environmental Health Perspectives journal published a study that revealed people who are exposed to two particular common pesticides are 2.5 times more likely to develop Parkinson's disease or Alzheimer's disease (EHP).

Even worse, the National Academy of Science estimates that cancer can be caused by pesticide residues. The allowable pesticide residual amounts in foods are now estimated to cause between 4,000 and 20,000 cases of cancer each year (WPL).

The fact is that the Environmental Protection Agency controls will not protect you and your family. Another problem is food additives. Food additives are found in most packaged food products. Companies use food additives to further shelf life. Food additives are used to make food look, smell, and taste just the way the customer likes it. The main goal for these big companies is profitability with no thought of the damage food additives may cause.

One of the most common additives in food is BHA. It looks like a waxy solid and used for animal feed, packaging, cosmetics, rubber, and also petroleum. The state of California has determined the danger it poses to human health, and has listed it as a carcinogen. However, today the additive is found in every packaged food we feed our families, even though it is known to cause Cancer! (Yoquinto)

13

How about genetically modified foods? Did you know that 90% of US corn has been genetically modified? But you don't know which, because the US Government doesn't require that food companies label their products as genetically modified. Honestly, we have no idea if what you're eating is a natural product or not. The biggest producer of genetically modified corn is Monsanto. And in 2012, Gilles-Eric Séralini and his colleagues from the University of Caen created a storm. A two-year Study concluded that rats fed genetically modified corn developed tumors, and also suffered from premature liver failure and kidney damage. They also died earlier than rats that were not given GMO foods. If everyone knew how much these chemicals damage the body there would be complete outrage from every family on this planet (Reuters).

One such GMO component is Xenoestrogens and it is everywhere. This element is in plastics, cosmetics, hair products, toothpastes, perfumes, metal cans, and many other products. Xenoestrogens bleed out of these products into liquids, foods, and containers, holding these products. After seeping out, they go into the human digestive system, and finally head for the other tissues and organs. They can also permeate out from the skin, when we use perfume or other cosmetic products. What exactly is the problem? Xenoestrogens mimic the role of estrogen and will cause hormone imbalances when they enter our bodies — in both men and women (Wollams).

In 2006, A Danish researcher's report uncovered facts that revealed even low-level exposure to xenoestrogens can cause premature puberty in girls. Other facts in the report included an increased risk of cancer and decreased fertility (Maron).

Toxins are everywhere around us. Dangerous chemicals are in the air we breathe, the water we drink, the foods we eat, and the cosmetics we put on our skin. Our bodies are under constant assault from chemicals that should not even be in our environment. Our bodies have evolved to take such chemicals, leaving us physically worn out, drained, and sick.

Here are the Facts:
Our bodies are geared to clear all toxins out and maintain and protect itself. However, with the fast pace of today, there are simply too many toxins to take in over and over again. We are getting toxins from every direction. It's just too much for our liver to cleanse properly. This is the reason many times we feel lethargic and continue to struggle with daily tasks everyday all day.

With continued health problems and stubborn fat, the bottom line is that our bodies were not made to digest all these artificial ingredients and poisons. That's why it's not coping. And it's this chronic toxicity that's behind most of the poor health people experience. A buildup of artificial elements will leave the body feeling lifeless and exhausted.

What if I eat organic foods and stick to a healthy diet?
It will help but only for short term. It is simply not enough just to eat healthy. Years and years of built up toxins and residue from poisons is still trapped within our bodies and leaking into every inch of your body. This infects tissues and muscles. It must all be eliminated and these toxins must be removed. The idea is to delete, reset, and start over.

Most formulas to detox may damage your health. Detox pills, organic lemonades, or herbal shakes may flush toxins from the body but only for a little while. Most detoxes provide no nutritional value and leave you nutrient deficient. We must detoxify and get rid of all toxins, while filling our bodies with vitamins and minerals during the process. The detoxes found today are just not sustainable, so it is easy to give up on them.

The truth is there is only one way to detox the body safely, while leaving precious vitamins and minerals behind to cleanse your cells with nutrition. Before I dive into the details, let me first tell you about the Ancient Health and Wellness Awesome Kernel

Mix (http://amzn.to/2DTKNdw). First, you will feel great after eating these kernels. They will leave precious nutrients and vitamins behind to sustain you for a good period. You will be eating good wholesome food that will leave you satisfied and feeling great, while getting rid of psoriasis. Most importantly, it's not expensive. Don't waste any more time looking for special ingredients because our body is craving nutrition. This program requires only 2 meals, common foods and ingredients that are well known, inexpensive, and easy-to-find at our website.

Do not be fooled by other bean mixes, which offer a great variety, but no beneficial nutrients combined. This mix has a purpose, and that purpose is beautiful skin and life longevity. We have now joined with Stealth Health Products to develop the Awesome Kernel Mix (http://amzn.to/2DTKNdw) to make this the most nutritional combination of kernels. Like elements in medication, these kernels are especially combined to deliver the most nutrients and give you beautiful skin in return. This combination not only results in beautiful skin, but promotes many other health benefits listed later on in this book, so please read on.

CHAPTER 4: INFLAMMATION

MORE THAN YOU THINK ABOUT PSORIASIS

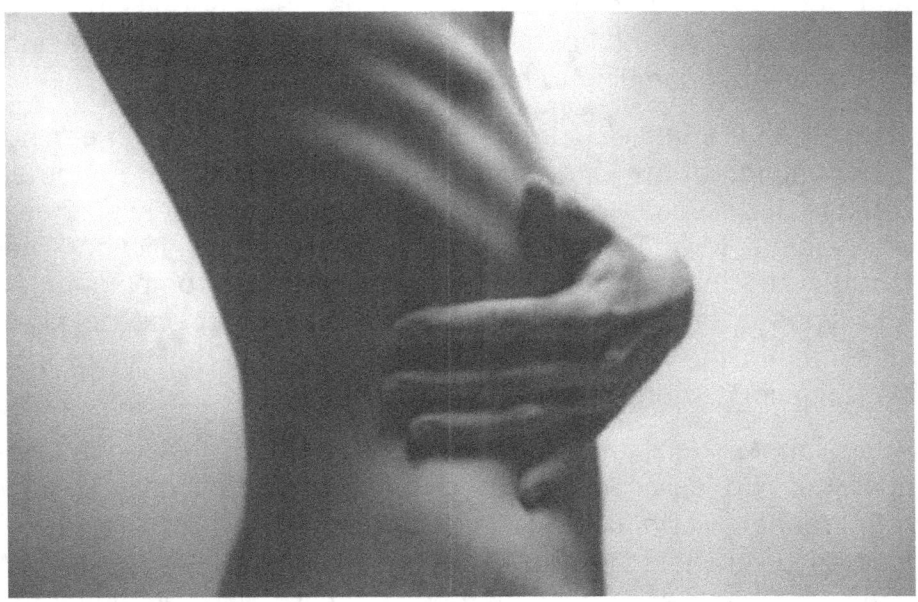

Inflammation is a natural process of repairing cell or tissue damage caused by physical injury. The underlying cause of inflammation is toxicity, infections, allergies, nutritional deficiencies or excess, injuries, and emotional trauma. Inflammation occurs when damaged tissue needs repair. As we get older, our immune system becomes more sensitive and our digestive juices do not tear apart food so effectively. As a consequence, food that is not digested properly will therefore become allergens. An allergen is a substance that causes a reaction within the body. This allows your body to retain water in an attempt to flush the allergen out of your system. This causes inflammation.

Inflammation and scaling of the skin affects 2-3% of the population. Dead skin cells pile up on the surface of our bodies, in our scalp, face, legs, elbows, lower back, palms, fingers and soles of our feet. This inflammation called psoriasis becomes patches of thick and red areas on our body that begin to look like plaques. These plaques of dead skin cells feel very sore and itch all the time. Psoriasis and psoriatic arthritis can go hand in hand. Arthritis and psoriasis are agonizing and limiting conditions that combine to make psoriatic arthritis.

The word "arthritis" originates from the Greek meaning "inflammation of the joint, "and is normally a reaction to internal disease. It causes severe pain, swelling, and ultimately stiffness of the joints. Millions of Americans suffer with this affliction. The fact is that arthritis is not a single condition, but a combination of 150 types of arthritis conditions, which can affect one or more joints within the body. Psoriatic arthritis is a huge part of this classification (Arthritis Foundation).

Approximately six million Americans struggling through the agony of psoriasis, one million of these are additionally coping with psoriatic arthritis. Psoriatic arthritis is a skin condition marked by a rapid buildup of rough, dry, dead skin cells that form thick scales. Psoriasis and arthritis (two autoimmune problems) occur when your body's immune system, which normally fights harmful organisms such as viruses and bacteria, begins to attack healthy cells and tissues. This abnormal immune response causes inflammation in joints.

When psoriasis occurs, the body's defense system is out of whack. Dry lesions begin to appear at the surface of the skin and begin to multiply vigorously. The itching and discomfort alone can literally make you ill. From the scalp to the elbows, psoriasis takes over. Outbreaks are natural occurrences and the results are devastating for the sufferer. Along with the physical side effects, the victim of this disease begins to feel alone, and distant towards co-workers and friends. Could this be inherited? Could it be a particular gene in your body that is causing this?

Well, both can be true. The horrible itching and soreness that comes with psoriasis can be caused by many things including overheating. Plaque psoriasis is the most common type of psoriasis. Outbreaks can start out small and get very bad within days. People who have no knowledge of psoriasis tend to be distant from people that do have psoriasis because they think it may be contagious. Psoriasis is not contagious. Along with these irritating physical side effects is the emotional factors. To compensate, psoriasis sufferers often wear pants and long sleeves to cover their skin, even in summer heat, and some avoid a social life altogether. It happened to me, so I know firsthand. I wore long sleeves and long pants only to sweat which caused my psoriasis to get worse. Doctors continually state that there is no known cure for psoriasis, only the hope to control its' severity. ***We do have a cure, however, so read on***. Each case of psoriasis is different, and may require a certain form of treatment or a combination of treatments to obtain relief. Most of those treatments available now work to lessen the redness and itching, but some tend to be harmful to internal organs or skin.

1st TIPS OF THE DAY

Get a quick boost of de-inflammation by combining any black tea you buy with just a little turmeric, not much. Feel the difference super quick and do it often.

Receding Gums?

Use one of the methods below to keep gums clean and bacteria free. Brushing teeth before bedtime is necessary because bacteria in the mouth accumulates at night. Use the tips below to brush teeth during the day and before bedtime.

1. Cut Aloe Vera in thin short slices and put in your mouth at night to heal gums while you sleep. This is also good for painful or inflamed gums from tooth decay.

2. Mix one-part licorice powder (http://amzn.to/2s5So1T) with one-part sesame seed oil. Mix into a paste. Now brush your teeth with it. This cleans the grit buildup on gums and teeth while preventing tartar buildup. There is an element in licorice (http://amzn.to/2s5So1T) that also helps prevent bacteria in the mouth and helps with receding gums to repair damage.

3. Brush teeth with a turmeric paste twice a day. Mix turmeric powder (whttp://amzn.to/2toDho7) with water to make a paste and brush teeth with it twice a day. Helps heal inflamed gums and prevent sores from bacteria buildup.

Another Recipe

Black Tea/Turmeric/Ginger, wait 30 minutes and add a small amount of coconut oil. Combine to make a hot tea. This is good to keep inflammation down throughout the body.

CHAPTER 5: KERNELS, A LIFE SAVER WITH PSORIASIS

THE ANCIENTS USED FOR HEALTH AND BEAUTIFUL SKIN

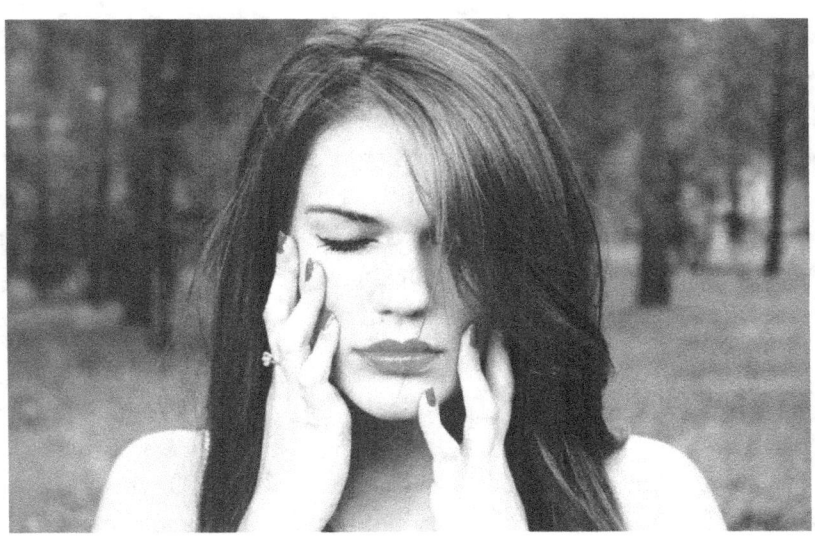

The Ancient Health and Wellness Awesome Kernel Mix (http://amzn.to/2DTKNdw) is what we call our New Product Kernels, which is an ancient food source that has been known to mankind for a very long time. With the right combination of kernels, you can receive great benefits. We know because we have tried it, and our families are healthy. We found out that the most nutritional, beneficial, and best tasting kernels can be put together with great health benefits as a result. Everybody is talking about eating seeds and nuts to live a longer, healthier life. Well, these are the seeds they are talking about. We know to always eat almonds for better health, but nobody mentions what type of seeds to eat. Here they are. Check out our website and order the Health and Wellness Awesome Kernel Mix (http://amzn.to/2DTKNdw) today! You will thank us later, We'll be here. We take pride in our product and only supply the freshest product to better serve our customers. Freshness and Satisfaction guaranteed. The cultivation of kernels is as old as early agriculture. It provides lots of health benefits, which include the following:

Good for Muscle Generation

Our organs and muscles need a constant supply of protein for repair and growth of healthy cells. Kernels, especially sprouted kernels, contain all the essential amino acids that are needed for good muscle-building and smooth functioning of the body. Visit our website to find recipes that show you how to make this little healthy meal delicious. You will receive a constant supply of protein eating this Awesome Kernel Mix (http://amzn.to/2DTKNdw) combination. The taste is excellent in soups, alone, or a side dish.

Controls Diabetes

Studies have shown that dietary fiber was found to be high in the case of the legume family. Kernels, along with beans and peas, belong to the legume family. Dietary fiber found food such as kernels help in controlling blood sugar levels. Dietary fiber slows down the rate at which food is absorbed by the blood and thus maintains the sugar level consistently.

Improves Digestion

As kernels contain high levels of dietary fiber, it improves digestion if consumed regularly. It also helps in easy bowel movement, resulting in decreased constipation.

Heart Health

Kernels, with their insignificant amounts of fat, are an ideal source of protein without adding any extra fat to the body, thereby promoting a healthy heart. Kernels contain magnesium, which helps in relaxing cardiovascular muscles and helping to lower blood pressure.

Prevents Atherosclerosis

Research conducted by the Department of Cereal and Foods Sciences in North Dakota showed that the consumption of kernels provides a supply of antioxidants that decreased the chances of developing atherosclerosis. Also, these antioxidants play a role in neutralizing free radicals and thereby preventing cell and gene damage (aging). (Sprout People)

Counteracting Cancer

Studies have shown that plant lectins, a separate type of plant protein originating from foods like kernels, wheat, peanuts, peas, and soy beans have a significant control factor over cancer cells. Research studies have shown that these lectins cause cytotoxicity and apoptosis, which means that they have a huge potential to control cancer growth.

Good Source of Folic Acid

Kernels are a good source of Vitamin B-complex, which contains folate or folic acid. The consumption of folic acid by pregnant woman helps in preventing birth defects. A lack of folic acid often results in neural tube defects. Folate found in kernels help in the formation of red blood cells, is good for pregnant women, and plays a key role in maintaining Vitamin B6 and Vitamin B12 levels. It is also known to be effective against hypertension and DNA damage, which may result in cancer.

Weight Management

Research studies suggest that the regular consumption of kernels can help in weight control and increase satiety (a state of being full when you eat).

Healthy Nervous System

It was long believed that micronutrients such as vitamins and minerals did not have an effect on the functioning of the brain. However, further research suggested that for the proper functioning of the brain, vitamins and minerals are equally important. Vitamins and minerals found in kernels are helpful for optimum brain functioning.

High Iron Content

Kernels contain high amounts of iron, which is needed by the body for optimal hemoglobin health (a red protein responsible for delivering oxygen to the blood). Approximately 36% of the iron of the Daily Recommended Value (DRV) comes from eating 1 cup (200 grams) of kernels every day.

Like anything else, at first to get rid of psoriasis, eat kernels until you see change and improvement, then eat once a week for optimal health. Once you see the great value in eating this great food, you will see the clearing up of your psoriasis. You can eat it at any time after that; just to clear any undigested food left in your intestines.

People with gallstones should avoid eating kernels due to too much fiber can build up too quickly depending on their metabolism. Otherwise, in order to get rid of built up medications, stress, and foods within the body, this is the sure proven way to see improvement not only in getting rid of psoriasis, but great improvement in your energy level, easy weight control, and overall good health. No more doctor visits with high bill costs, unless of course, you have a cold, in which medication like antibiotics will do the trick. If people would only try this, it would certainly be an important part of their meals. Everyone would eat kernels if they knew all the health benefits they contain. The ultimate result by eating these kernels: better thinking, calmer mind, easy flow of body movement, and many other amazing things. Who would even consider what such a simple small meal can do. I did not, until I was forced to research. I had no choice. When I found what these kernels could do, I was amazed and you will be amazed too.

Natural and Easy Detox for the Body

Your whole life can change for the better with one simple meal. It is really hard to believe how simple this is. It took me years and years to find this, and like you, I was looking for a more complicated answer, until finally I gave up, let the doctors deal with me, and started taking medications that made me swell and damaged my liver. After feeling I wanted to die, I began to study again, and remembered my classes in Biotechnology, and said to myself, "I can do this."

For the Ancient Aztec Health and Wellness Mix, even if you only eat a single teaspoon, one can detox the body. Immediately after swallowing a teaspoon, you will see a miracle happen. No more worries. You should feel lighter physically in about 1-4 hours depending on how bad your body needs detoxing. The combination of kernels actually speaks to your cells by electronic signals to let go of toxins. After detoxing the body, these kernels leave behind serious nutrients and minerals that your body absolutely needs to survive and thrive. Unlike other detox methods, which deplete the body of nutrients and minerals, leave the body thirsting for water and dangerous dehydration, these kernels purify the body while leaving nutrients behind. Don't believe me? Try this natural remedy for psoriasis and watch how these little miniature mini-me kernels figure out the problem. I mean, why not? I learned and studied these in detail. I made A's in Biotechnology. I just did not have the confidence to research myself and figure it out, simple as that. When I discovered the magic of these kernels and then began to combine them for their particular nutritional value, it was like a miracle. My skin cleared up, my mind cleared up, and my body cleared up. In my research, these kernels not only give signals to your cells to eliminate toxins, but grab the toxins themselves and prepare for elimination. Amazing, right?

25

Who can believe that these kernels could do that? The Indians and Romans that lived until 150-500 years old did, that's who.

We have researched kernels for years and have come up with a great tasting medley everyone will love. Usually, kernels, to put it lightly, taste like crap, but because we are dedicated cooks, we have developed the Awesome Kernel Mix (http://amzn.to/2DTKNdw) combination that tastes good and everyone in the family can enjoy. Any illness, including hangovers from food poisoning; this combination of kernels, just eating only ONE teaspoon of the soup created from cooking these kernels, can eliminate hangover from any food poisoning after or even during the sickness, with miraculous and quick results. Our kernels eliminate toxic free radicals in the body because they are specially combined by nutrient quantity to provide the most valuable minerals and vitamins while tasting great. After eating the Ancient Aztec Health and Wellness Awesome Kernel Mix (http://amzn.to/2DTKNdw), you are going to have more time now without this horrible affliction; it's time to look great and find something that looks great on you to show off that beautiful skin. We hear you, because we have been there. We suffered with afflictions of bad childhood, super stressful situations in life, and now we are older. We feel you and your heart. We wrote this book to help you see how to get healthy the easiest and cheapest way with great results. You don't have to spend a lot of money to be healthy, but you have to be well informed. This book informs you of the truth; the truth about psoriasis and how to heal. No longer does Psoriasis have to be a part of your life. Now...... Now, live and you will never have to look at the word "Psoriasis" again. God bless you.

Something also very important to know about eating these kernels is that once you eat them, and see a difference in your well-being, you can stop eating them altogether until you feel you need to eat them again. The protein supplied by eating these magical kernels builds up in your body and will continuously protect your cells from toxins. Everyone is different internally, so you may need to eat these kernels more or less often after the clearing of psoriasis, it just depends on your individual situation. Another thing to mention, you will see that you can eat all the things you could not eat before, and still feel well. After starting your <u>Awesome Kernel Mix</u> regimen, just monitor how you feel, and eat the kernels when you see fit. They will work again to take all the toxins out of your body, even if you eat one teaspoon. Wonderful- right? Yes.

Go to our website for a full description of the benefits of our <u>Awesome Kernel Mix</u>. It is so important if you take any medication at all to avoid build up, something doctor's never talk about or warn their patients about. Buildup of medication causes human suffering, inflammation, and always leads to deterioration of the body which can be fatal. These natural kernels in combination, sort of like medication, will pack a powerful punch. Just a few of the many nutrients in our kernels are listed below:

230 calories
18g protein
15g of fiber
3.5g sugar
>1g fat
358 ml folate (90 percent DRV)
1 ml manganese (49 percent DRV)
6.6 ml iron (37 percent DRV)
356 ml phosphorus (36 percent DRV)
0.5 ml copper (25 percent DRV)
0.5 ml thiamine (22 percent DRV)
731 ml potassium (21 percent DRV)
71 ml magnesium (18 percent DRV)
0.4 ml vitamin B6 (18 percent DRV)
2.5 ml zinc (17 percent DRV)
1.3 ml vitamin B5 (13 percent DRV)

Go to our website to find out all the minerals and nutrients our kernels provide. We have some great recipes also.

Kernels are a natural and vegan way to get these vitamins and minerals in your system quickly. Fructose covering found in many vitamins bought at your local store will ever be on these naturally grown kernels. There will never be side effects from eating these naturally nutritious little seeds. The vitamins listed above and many more minerals listed on our website will remain in your body until you eat kernels again. That is very good for your body's supplemental needs.

The Information against Beans (not Kernels)

The paleo diet actually states that people should not eat beans. However, the benefits far outweigh the negatives. It is important to check with your doctor before you eat beans or any food you may have concerns about.

1. Beans and digestion (the musical fruit).

Beans and kernels must be properly soaked, drained, boiled. You can boil beans in a slow boil. Beans can make you pass gas more.

Special Note: What is important to note here is that methane is the result of a toxic environment. If eating beans or lentils causes gas, it is because the body has too much toxicity combined with a buildup of water. When using the Awesome Kernel Mix, your body is trying to decrease water, therefore you may have to release what is necessary to begin the detox process. Know that this is temporary, and after your body decreases water content, you will be back to normal with no buildup of gas at all. You will find your stomach begin to flatten out after all the water and gas is gone. This build up was caused by stress and toxicity that was not dealt with for an extended period.

2. Beans can irritate autoimmune diseases.

Legumes, beans, peas, peanuts, tofu, and soy milk all contain lectins, and can irritate IBS. When combined with other ailments such as Type

2 Diabetes, allergies, sclerosis, peptic ulcers, Crohn's disease, and arthritis; lectins can exasperate IBS.

3. Beans have plenty of carbohydrates and starch.

Beans are a starchy food, high in carbohydrates. Eating significant amounts of Beans (not kernels) may interfere with weight loss. This has never been proven.

4. Beans (not kernels) consist of week estrogen mimics

Estrogen mimics interfere with hormone function. Soy beans and fava beans provide phytoestrogens. Phytoestrogens have always been in plants and act as a defense system within the plant to keep predators away. It disrupts the reproductive system of the predator. The Red Clover plant has been known to have phytoestrogens that do just this (Axe).

Factually, we do not believe the evidence against beans. We have found that eating these special legumes in combination is great for health and skin. The Ancient Health and Wellness Awesome Kernel Mix is natural, wholesome, and works. Besides, you do not have to eat it all the time, once it is built up in your body you only need to eat these kernels when you have a breakout of psoriasis, which may be once a month, once every 3 months or even once a year. You may not get a breakout for some time but these kernels help with gentle detox for your body if you want to use them for a short period. That is what is so great and special about the Ancient Health and Wellness Awesome Kernel Mix (http://amzn.to/2DTKNdw). Only we have combined these special kernels to deliver the greatest benefit to our friends and psoriasis sufferers. You will immediately see a difference in body aches, fatigue, and many other symptoms and ailments. It has been tested by several members of our family and staff for several years before we wrote this book.

The Information in Support of Beans

1. Beans are extremely potent in protein and fiber. If you are vegan, beans provide a great amount of protein. If you're on a diet, beans provide a sense of fullness that can result in less eating.

2. Beans provide a consistent fountain of glucose for energy. Sugar, corn syrup, or agave nectar, which includes fructose, can be associated with gaining belly fat, increased risk of heart disease, higher LDL levels, and poor insulin sensitivity. Since sugar is half glucose and half fructose. We recommend eliminating fructose entirely (except on cheat days), and instead using legumes as a carbohydrate source. Beans contain starch which breaks down into glucose. Too much glucose can make subcutaneous fat under the skin. Fat under the skin is not associated with disease as much as abdominal fat. Legumes provide steady energy to the body without adding abdominal fat. However, switching from a high-carb diet to a low-carb diet quickly may result in energy crashes. Your system needs a few weeks to adjust to different kinds of foods that provide fuel for the body.

3. Beans are high magnesium, copper, selenium, molybdenum, manganese, iron, folate, and has many antioxidants. Beans are for sure not nutritionally empty. Depending on the legume, beans can provide decent amounts of vitamins and many minerals.

Any elements in beans and legumes like anti-nutrients, lectins, and phytic acid can easily be drained out when soaking beans. Most of these can be cooked out leaving very beneficial vitamins and nutrients behind. Soaking works in leaving phytic acid behind and boiling beans reduces lectin levels. It is best to boil beans instead of slow-cooking them. Slow-cooked kidney beans and red beans, usually used in chili, can lead to lectin poisoning. There are dozens of cases of lectin poisoning in the U.S. every year.

4. Beans are related in reduced risk of colon cancer.

Beans and kernels can reduce the risk of colorectal cancer. This disease is common and just as dangerous as lung cancer. This is a pretty good reason to consider eating legumes.

One study about colon polyps found that people who ate beans or kernels were far less likely to develop precancerous tumors or polyps. One clinical trial over a four-year period concluded that 2,000 adults who ate beans or legumes had fewer cancerous polyps and less cancer. How interesting that the same study notes that people who ate fruits and vegetables did not get the same benefits as given by lentils. Legumes have anti-inflammatory and anticancer properties and act to prevent cancer in other ways. When digested, the carbs in legumes are broken down by our gut flora into a fatty acid called butyrate, which acts with various phytonutrients to prevent cancer and add anti-inflammatory properties (Axe).

With the pros and cons listed here, you decide. This book is written in belief that kernels are far better for you. Benefits of lentils have been proven throughout the centuries. Just by looking at what the Ancient Aztec Indians ate that allowed them to live 150 years. Tim Ferriss, one of the richest men in the world, swears by lentils as a go-to-meal to keep healthy and live long (Moyer). In Ancient Times, Indians and Romans and Biblical populations lived a very long time with no illnesses. Only this combination of lentils provided at our website will give you a multiple boost of great energy. Like medications that have several elements to alleviate illness, so does the combination of specific Awesome Kernel Mix that we provide. Go to our website now and order your Awesome Kernel Mix Today! Everyone that has tried our Health and Wellness Awesome Kernel Mix has been satisfied and very grateful we have supplied this product to the public. Try it and see. The Awesome Kernel Mix is very inexpensive for the benefits these special little kernels deliver. It will literally change your life and the way you feel within days. I spent thousands of dollars over a lifetime with doctor visits and medication that only made me sicker. Once built up in your body's system, there is no need to eat these magical kernels every week, but every other week or even once a month. You will see the difference in your health, skin, and overall wellbeing. It certainly changed my life.

CHAPTER 6: **CHICKEN**

A STAPLE AT THE TABLE FOR HEALING

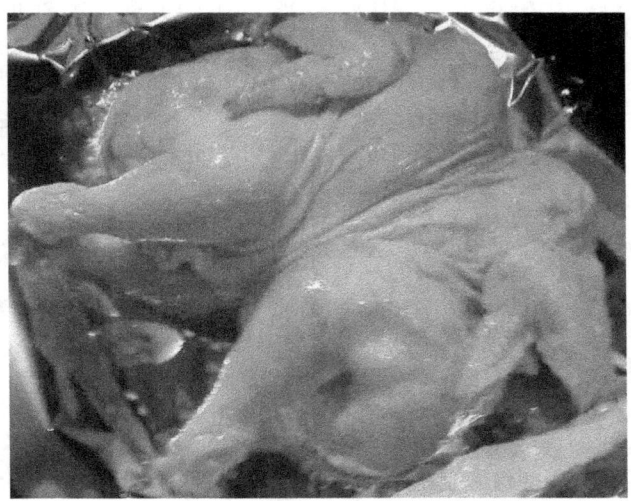

Please go to our website to see an important video on how to cut Spatchcock Chicken.

We want you to get rid of Psoriasis, which is our goal. We deal with suppliers that only do business with high end restaurants to get the freshest spices available. Our families are important to us, so only the best, freshest spices and herbs will do. Order your spices and herbs at our website.

This recipe includes herbs that you need to keep healthy and happy throughout your lifetime. Like medications that have many elements in them, spices and herbs combined can create a big benefit health wise. It's called Spatchcock Chicken, which is a way of cutting a chicken. Baste chicken at least once while cooking to allow spices to penetrate chicken. Use the spices mentioned below together or alternate them together. Ginger and Coriander together is a must for a good foundation. Then combine the rest at different times. Mustard kernels and Cardamom kernels crushed together make a killer lemon-pepper flavoring, so use it. Combine these with Ginger and Coriander. Then, use Mustard kernels and Cardamom kernels and alternate with Turmeric powder (http://amzn.to/2toDho7) which is available fresh on our website or use the amazon link provided. We make sure to choose the freshest spices for the best price. Please go to our website and order your fresh spices and herbs today! Powder form is the most convenient and best way to take advantage of the benefits of spices at your fingertips! Go to our website at https://nurseoasis.com/spices-to-your-liking and order today!

After cutting your chicken; add these spices on the skin:

- Ginger: we all want Ginger chicken, it tastes great

- Coriander (seeds)

- Lemon or salt and pepper to taste

- Turmeric (http://amzn.to/2toDho7) (optional) (Use pepper with Turmeric for better absorption)

- Mustard Kernels (alternate with turmeric) Crushed. Visit our website for more information and to get these spices at best quality if requested. Just order at the links for the Freshest Spices.

- Cardamom Kernels (alternate with turmeric) Crushed. Visit our website for more information and get these spices at best quality if requested. Just click link and order.

- Garlic Salt (optional)

- Soy Sauce (optional and choose your favorite: we use Kikkoman). We use this simply for extra flavor only.

- As a side dish, mix rice and water with a small amount of turmeric, butter, and salt to taste. This will complement the chicken nicely. Any spices you add, like oregano or cilantro will only make it better tasting. To Your Health!

- For a vegetable, cauliflower is good because it is easily digestible and contains good vitamins that again complement the chicken in taste and combined spices.

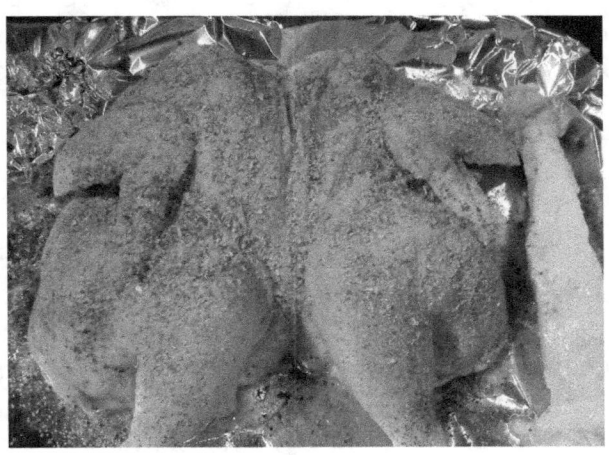

Please consult your doctor before using any of these spices just to make sure it does not interfere with any medication you may be taking.

Important NOTE: Try to realize that purchasing fresh spices in powder form can give you a huge advantage over everybody else in staying healthy. Spices at your fingertips allows you to quickly make a tea that benefits you for a lifetime. Go to our website now and order to prevent future diseases just by ordering spices you can combine later to cook with for a delicious meal or make a disease-fighting tea mixture. We have a great company we work with to bring our customers the freshest spices for the best price. This is prevention at its finest!

Using a wide space to administer these spices like the Spatchcock Chicken way is best. By cutting the chicken and laying it flat, you can add these spices to the skin of the chicken, yes, I said the skin, and do not worry about cholesterol right now. We are going to use the skin to eat in order to delve into our digestive system. Of course, you can remove the skin from the chicken and just add the spices on top without the skin. By eating these spices in combination, it will travel through the roadway of your intestines, giving signals to your body, telling your cells to prepare to eliminate toxins. We have studied Biotechnology and the digestive tract in detail and know what we are talking about. Try it, and you will see a great improvement in not only your skin, but overall energy and health. Let's not forget scalp psoriasis; you can forget you ever had it with the Ancient Aztec Health and Wellness Awesome Kernel Mix or the Spatchcock Chicken meal prepared with herbs listed above. Remember, watch the "How to Cut Spatchcock Chicken" on our website After watching the video, cut chicken when completely defrosted for easier handling, and use the complete chicken with a huge surface area to put all these spices and pour them on. Not only will your chicken taste great, but at the same time you will be eating something that prolongs your life, gets rid of psoriasis, helps prevent and sometimes remove cancer cells and toxins in the body, and by the way, is a natural detox. This meal may be eaten with any side dish (see our recipes at our website) for adults and children alike. At our website, we supply all the spices needed for this meal, because we want to make sure you get the freshest herbs and spices. We want you to get rid of Psoriasis, which is our goal.

You really cannot lose eating the Spatchcock Chicken meal. This meal is so simple, who would have thought a staple in a common American meal could be so beneficial? As for western medicine and American doctors, they may eat this meal themselves, but recommending it to their very own patients hurts their pocketbook. It is not beneficial for Western doctors to recommended easy healing remedies because getting you better is not in the plan. Keeping you buying medications that builds up in your body, and eventually kills you, is. The reason is simple: insurance companies pay big money for the medication you buy for psoriasis, and you ultimately pay for overpriced medications that do you more harm than good, all health care premiums, and copayments. That is the plan.

We reluctantly asked several big companies to sponsor us, for example, National Foundation of Psoriasis and many other sub-companies that dealt with National Foundation of Psoriasis, and some did not even email us back; others said simply, "We are not interested." However, they sure did go to our website to see their competition and how many views we were ranking. I'm talking about the worst companies in the world, how greedy and disgusting.

Special Note

Have Psoriasis in your Hair? Eat the Ancient Aztec Health and Wellness Awesome Kernel Mix (http://amzn.to/2DTKNdw) **and be free of this forever. Continue eating this mix until you see results, which should not take long.**

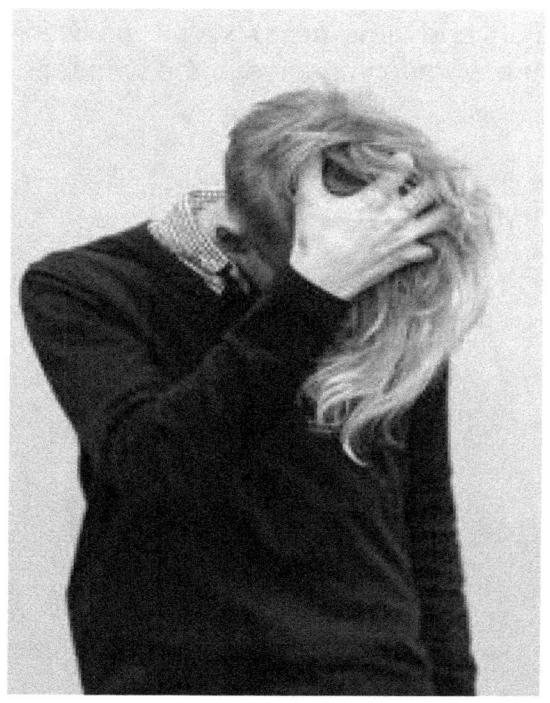

What is the best shampoo for scalp psoriasis?

You'd think it would be dandruff shampoo but that makes it worse. Herbal Essence (http://amzn.to/2s5Hjlp) **shampoo keeps hair and scalp clean. Use it regularly to keep flakes at bay. Go to** http://amzn.to/2s5Hjlp **to get this quickly. We have chosen the best for your hair.**

What is the best conditioner for scalp psoriasis?

Garnier Fructis (http://amzn.to/2t9LwUO) Sleek and Shine or 3 in 1 Conditioner. Either one will help take away any flaking left over from washing and rinsing. Wash hair with Herbal Essence and rinse with Fructis Conditioner (http://amzn.to/2t9LwUO). Combined, these two will clean your hair. Use regularly to maintain healthy hair with shine. Insert link shown into your browser and follow links to get these particular shampoo and conditioner quickly and start using for beautiful, shiny hair with no flakes. We have chosen the best for your hair.

CHAPTER 7: **MARSHMALLOW**

PSORIASIS AND THE MARSHMALLOW PLANT

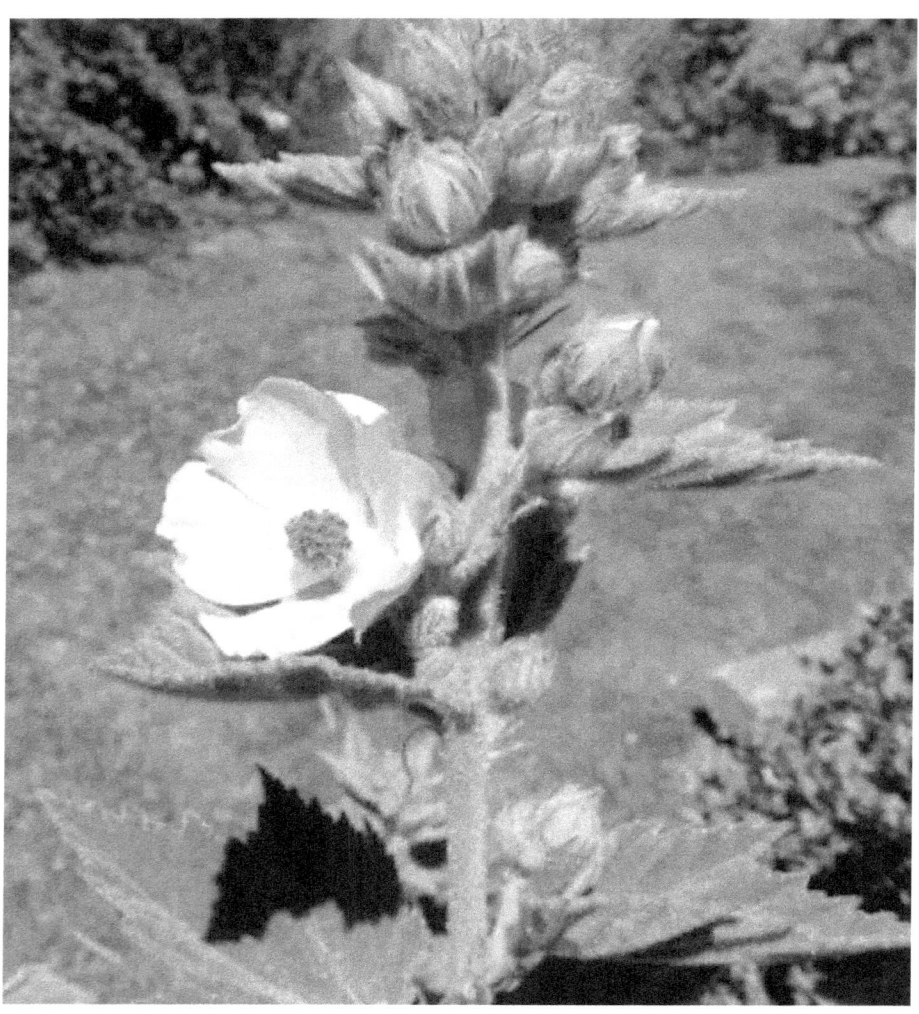

You can grow this plant super easy and the benefits are as follows:

1. If you have periodontal disease, which can be associated with long term psoriasis mild or chronic, stick the leaves in your mouth at night and keep it there until the morning. Even if you leave the leaves in your mouth for 30 minutes, it will help. This will tremendously decrease inflammation and allow for new gum growth.

2. Get a leaf and put it in your tea or coffee, this will help with any inflammation in the throat.

As with many things, do not use the leaf for an extended period, everything is moderation is great. You can order seeds at our website. This is a great company we buy seeds from that only sell heirloom, non-GMO seeds. If you need the seeds use a seed company you trust for heirloom seeds. Please go to our website to get the best seeds. We have done our research. The best heirloom seeds are at our website.

Marshmallow Plant and Benefits

1. Treatment for Coughs and Colds

For sore throat, colds, and coughs, marshmallow can be taken orally to reduce pain, swelling, and congestion. Marshmallow has cough suppressing properties for anyone suffering from a sore throat, cough or cold. It has the ability to protect mucus membranes and eliminate irritation in the throat. Marshmallow can reduce swelling in the lymph nodes, speed up healing time, and reduce painful dry coughing. Marshmallow is included in many cough syrups and throat lozenges. This proves it's one of the most potent natural cough remedies.

Marshmallow when combined with other anti-inflammatory or antibacterial herbs, natural oils for the throat, such as Echinacea, lemon, myrrh, oregano, cypress, or frankincense essential oils, works even better to alleviate pain. When these herbs are combined, they target bacteria and help with throat discomfort. This is a natural cure and targets the underlying cause of the sickness to ease discomfort.

2. Battles Bacterial Infections

Urinary tract infections, tonsillitis, bronchitis, and respiratory infections can all be managed by taking marshmallow root at the first sign of swelling, burning, or tenderness. Marshmallow helps with rapid healing by increasing the secretion of urine to increase release of toxins while naturally killing bacteria inside the urinary tract. That is why marshmallow is recommended for kidney stone symptoms.

3. Repairs the Gut Lining, Blocking Leaky Gut Syndrome

Research states that marshmallow is a great way to treat digestive disorders, including leaky gut syndrome. A leaky gut means there are tiny slits in the gut, which allows toxins to enter the bloodstream that can initiate autoimmune reactions. Marshmallow helps restore health to the gut lining by creating a protective layer around the slits and stop all leaking from the gut.

Studies show it is also beneficial for IBS, ulcerative colitis, and Crohn's disease.

4. Reduces Digestive Problems

Marshmallow can alleviate heartburn, stomach ulcer symptoms, constipation, and diarrhea. It relieves acid in the stomach and prevents stomach "burning." Marshmallow in tea form works and does not cause any side effects. The result is a soothing feeling for the stomach. This tea can be combined with peppermint or ginger for an even better result.

5. Heals Skin

Marshmallow is used to treat problems such as insect bites, wounds, burns, scrapes, dry skin, or peeling skin. This cool little plant is well tolerated by those with allergies and hypersensitive skin conditions. It can help provide major relief from itching, swelling, redness, and scrapes. Marshmallow has serious anti-irritant properties that kill bacteria. Helping to heal the nerve-sense system of the skin, marshmallow secretes mucilage, which is known to soften the skin and is often added to skin-care products and ointments. Studies also show it is beneficial to eczema and dermatitis. Marshmallow root acts as a skin buffer to help moisturize and protect very sensitive skin. Marshmallow root is found in lip balms, hair conditioners, sun protection products, and salves. If you can find an ointment made of marshmallow root, you can combine it with drops of coconut oil, tea tree oil, or Aloe Vera extract to have an even bigger impact.

6. Decreases Inflammation and Supports Heart Health

Heart disease is caused by acute and chronic inflammation. Marshmallow has anti-inflammatory properties that help the heart stay healthy. Marshmallow also has ant-ulcer, anti-lipidemic, and anti-cholesterol building properties with no side effects at all. Known to increase good cholesterol (HDL) within the body, it's time to grow this little plant or better yet, go get some tea at the health food store.

7. Alleviates Water Retention

Marshmallow acts like "water pills" that are taken to lower water retention, and reduce edema and bloated stomach. During PMS or menopause, Marshmallow can help increase urination and bring you back into balance (Axe).

Let's Define Marshmallow Root

Marshmallow has many benefits, but what exactly is it? It's a native plant to Africa and part of Europe that has been used as an herbal treatment for centuries. It used to be made into candy. It has a very long history in folk medicine that goes back more than 2000 years ago. It was used to treat coughs, sore throats, and congestion. Today, marshmallow is still used in holistic medicine the same way it was used many years ago. This plant has powerful ingredients to relieve and break up mucus, reduce inflammation, and kill bacteria with no side effects. This plant boosts immunity and prevents diseases around the world.

The young leaves of the marshmallow plant can be eaten raw, boiled in tea, or even fried. Drinking water with marshmallow allows the substance to form a protective coating around cell membranes. The plant's leaves and roots can be used and eaten.

Marshmallow also helps with swelling in nasal passages. It works to decrease swelling of the digestive system and promotes cell viability which protects our cells within the stomach lining.

Flavonoids in Marshmallow helps prevent damage within the body that can lead to disease, including cancerous tumor growth. It also helps speed up healing by removing damaged or dead cells from the body. All at once, marshmallow protects our cells through the combination of stages they go through, while getting rid of harmful cell adhesions that affect the growth of healthy cells (Axe).

Marshmallow Root and Medications

Since marshmallow coats and protects the lining of the stomach, it can interfere with the medications you are taking. If you are pregnant, nursing, or diagnosed with an existing condition, marshmallow root can alter the medication you are taking. Marshmallow can interfere with the way medications are absorbed. It is also possible for marshmallow to interfere with blood sugar control, so check with your doctor before using Marshmallow. Due to Marshmallow effects on water retention, you want to closely monitor blood sugar levels. Do not take marshmallow at least two weeks before a scheduled surgery (Axe). Always check with your doctor before starting any new regimen.

Drinking water is best when using Marshmallow root. This allows it to expand and protect cells. Experts suggest drinking Marshmallow at least one to two hours before or after using medications.

It also depends on how concentrated the supplement is. The exact dosage depends on your condition. Usually one to two teaspoons of powdered Marshmallow taken each day is effective and safe. Drinking tea all day will soothe a cough and reduce any built-up phlegm. Marshmallow can go with fennel, thyme, and honey for even greater benefits. Look for powder or teas online. We will post a link soon on our website. If making your own tea, it is best to purchase the powder or dried Marshmallow leaves. Steep leaves or powder in hot water.

Here are several ways to effectively use Marshmallow root in its different forms:

Capsules, tea, or powder can be used for leaky gut syndrome, Crohn's disease, ulcerative colitis, and IBS. In this case, a dosage of six grams daily is helpful. For dry skin, an ointment or balm with Marshmallow root can be applied to affected area.

Marshmallow Root Side Effects

Marshmallow has been around for centuries and is proven to be very safe. Backed by many years of use, Marshmallow only strengthens the body to fight infections. There have been no clinical trials on humans and few on animals. I guess the fact that it has been used for years makes it a go-to for healthy outcomes.

Marshmallow Root Takeaways

Marshmallow root can help treat leaky gut syndrome, bacterial infections, coughs and colds, digestive issues. It also helps with less water retention, healing of skin conditions, and supports heart health. The biggest benefit from Marshmallow is the fact that it protects membranes around our cells (Axe).

2nd TIP OF THE DAY

If you drink hot or cold beverages in the morning: Try adding a very small amount of turmeric in your drink, and/or marshmallow leaf (super easy to grow). This will deliver a quick inflammation resistant portion of wellbeing inside your body quickly. Turmeric tastes good in coffee, however, very little is needed and too much can overcome the coffee taste, so be careful. ⅛ a teaspoon is good for 1 cup of coffee or any drink cold or hot.

CHAPTER 8: GARDENING

GARDENING AND PSORIASIS: THE PLAIN AND SIMPLE FACT

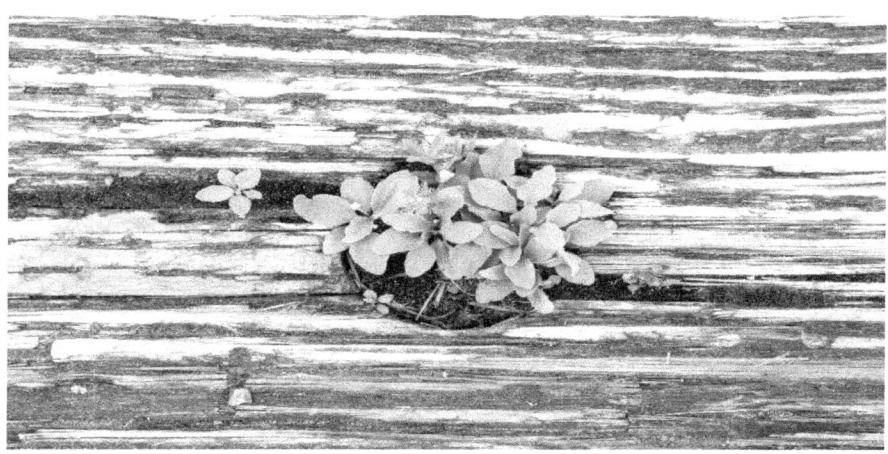

Emotional healing is the hardest thing to face because it is not tangible. Gardening can save your life every morning. Instead of putting on your running shoes, exchange it for garden boots and start mulching and planning for your new little garden. Composting should be made mandatory for every household so we can cut down on all landfills and heal our soil. Everyone needs to save their vegetable trimmings, eggshells, coffee grounds, and tea bags and put them into the compost which in turn goes back into the soil in your garden to help nourish the delicious food you're growing. Gardening can be life-changing sending you hunting for new recipes and boosting your veggie intake. It allows you to be in the moment for a moment.

To put it simply, gardening helps calm the mind, whether you're thinking about gardening or starting a small windowsill garden, the experience of eating your first fresh picked basil can be extremely rewarding. Growing vegetables can help your bank account, your mental well-being, your waistline, and your overall health. Gardening can help your children have skills and values they can carry with them forever. Starting small is important. The most important thing gardening can do is calm the mind. Look at different garden pictures on the internet just to begin to calm your mind. If you're tired of going to the gym or running down the block near your home, try starting a small garden or even a small pot on your windowsill. Looking and watching your plant grow will help calm the mind and relax the body and ultimately help in the elimination of your skin condition. Gardening is an important part of relaxation and calming the mind even if you do not grow anything. Just by walking in your garden or yard and looking at trees while thinking about something positive can help. It's important to know you are loved by the universe. I myself have no family, but I do have a creator. Believe that the universe is on your side for your better good. Slowing down mentally is a huge part of calming the mind which is absolutely required to help with skin conditions like psoriasis. I have spoken to many people that have mentioned to me that small gardening even in a small space can literally prepare the body for detox. All these reasons given above is enough to say that gardening, no matter how small, can be a big benefit when trying to heal a skin condition like psoriasis.

Below are some simple plants you can grow in a very small garden that will benefit your wellbeing for a lifetime:

You're Small Garden Needs These (easy to grow)

Aloe Vera

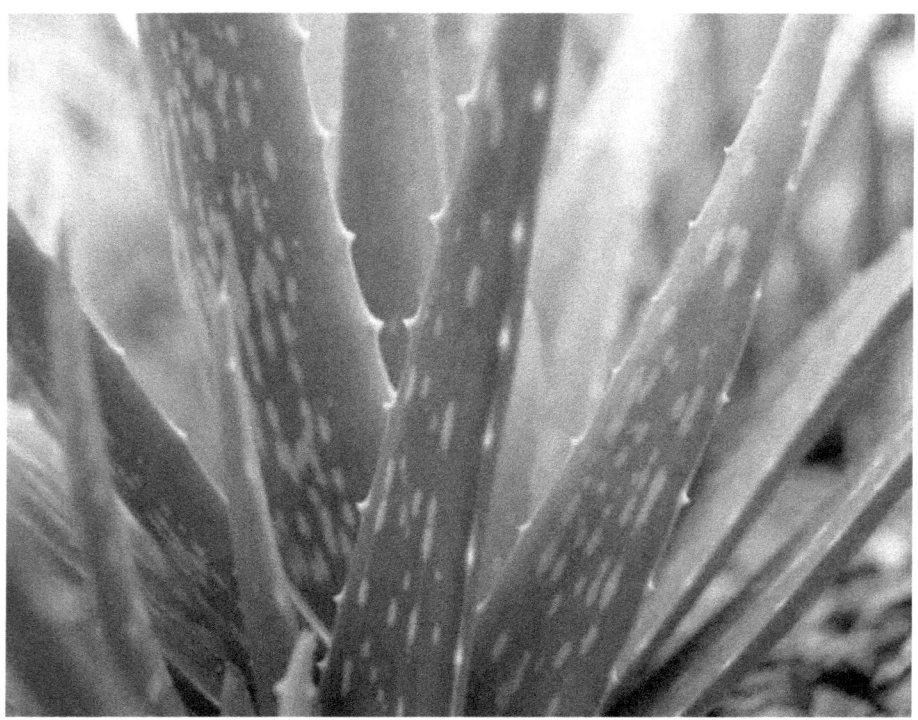

The Aloe Vera grows with well drained dry or moist soil. It needs sun but can grow anywhere. Even though the taste is not for everyone, it can be eaten. The sap from this little plant expedites healing and reduces infections for many things. It helps with burns, wounds, cuts, eczema, digestive problems, and poor appetite. By drinking the juice, it can treat ulcerative colitis, and chronic constipation. Please visit our website for heirloom seeds. We research the best seeds for the lowest cost.

Why is the Aloe Plant Important to a Psoriasis Sufferer?

1. Remove Makeup: Aloe Vera offers cooling properties that calm the skin.
2. Hair Conditioner: Simply massage a small amount of Aloe Vera gel an let it work for about two minutes before rinsing it off.
3. Shampoo-Enhancer: Adding a small amount of Aloe Vera to your shampoo makes the hair shinier and healthier.

4. Increase Hair Growth: Aloe Vera is packed with an enzyme which is known to stimulate hair growth.

5. Treat Acne: Due to its ability to reduce inflammation, Aloe Vera is very effective in treating acne.

6. Prevent and Eliminate Stretch Marks: Aloe Vera possesses regenerative properties, which help both prevent and remove stretch marks.

7. Heal Sunburns: Thanks to its antiseptic properties, this ancient plant is extremely effective in healing sunburns.

8. Skin-Moisturizer: By supplying the cells with oxygen, Aloe Vera helps strengthen skin tissue and moisturize its texture.

9. Treat Herpes, Eczema, psoriasis, Dermatitis, and other Skin Allergies: Aloe Vera has the ability to penetrate deeply into the skin layers, which helps treat conditions like herpes, psoriasis, dermatitis, and other skin allergies.

10. Personal Lubricant: As already mentioned above, it works as an effective moisturizer.

11. Shaving gel: Thanks to its anti-inflammatory and soothing properties, it gives a smooth surface, without the common irritation and redness.

12. Strengthen your nails: Aloe Vera helps *strengthen* the *nails* and heal damaged beds and cuticles. You can either soak the nails in Aloe Vera Juice or massage them with Aloe Vera Gel.

13. Swollen Gums: Again, its soothing properties soothe swollen gums, while optimizing body`s defense mechanisms. All you have to do is to apply it onto the affected area.

14. Ease Menstrual Cramps: Using Aloe Vera juices orally helps ease menstrual cramps, reduce fatigue, and alleviate pain.

15. Fight the Flu and Colds: As discussed in the very beginning, Aloe Vera has a robust nutritional profile and is packed with numerous vitamins, minerals, and amino acids, all of which work together to strengthen the immune system and protect against flu and colds.

Note: Only use Aloe Vera Externally. If you use Aloe Vera Internally, the gel is the only thing you want to put between teeth and gums that are inflamed or swollen. Visit our blog for more information on the side effects of the Aloe Vera Plant Latex by going to https://nurseoasis.com/aloe-vera-plant-means, then click on more information, and go to Aloe Vera Side effects to find out more.

Marshmallow Plant

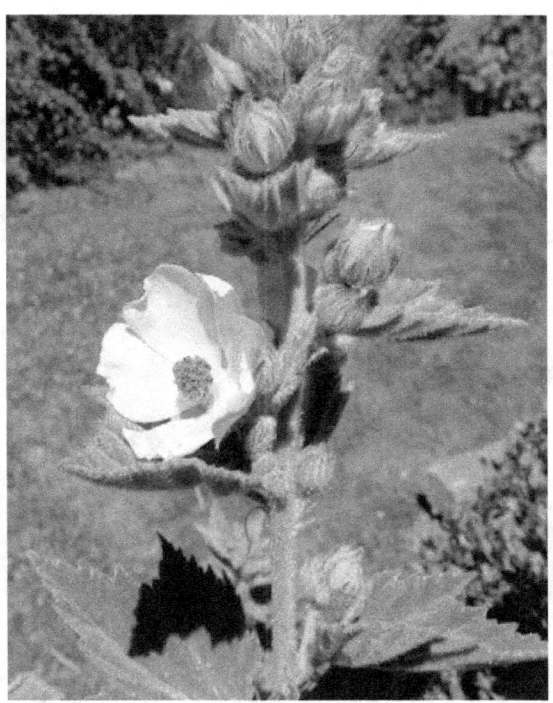

Prepared as a tea, marshmallow can get rid of excess stomach acid, help with inflammations and irritations of the urinary tract, treat swollen respiratory mucus membranes, treat peptic ulcerations, insect bites, bruises, skin inflammations, relieve gastritis, reduce stomach acid, and many other ailments. This plant can be taken internally or used externally. It can even be used to treat splinters. The leaves can be added to salads and eaten or boiled to make a tea. Please visit our website for heirloom seeds. We research the best seeds for the lowest cost.

:

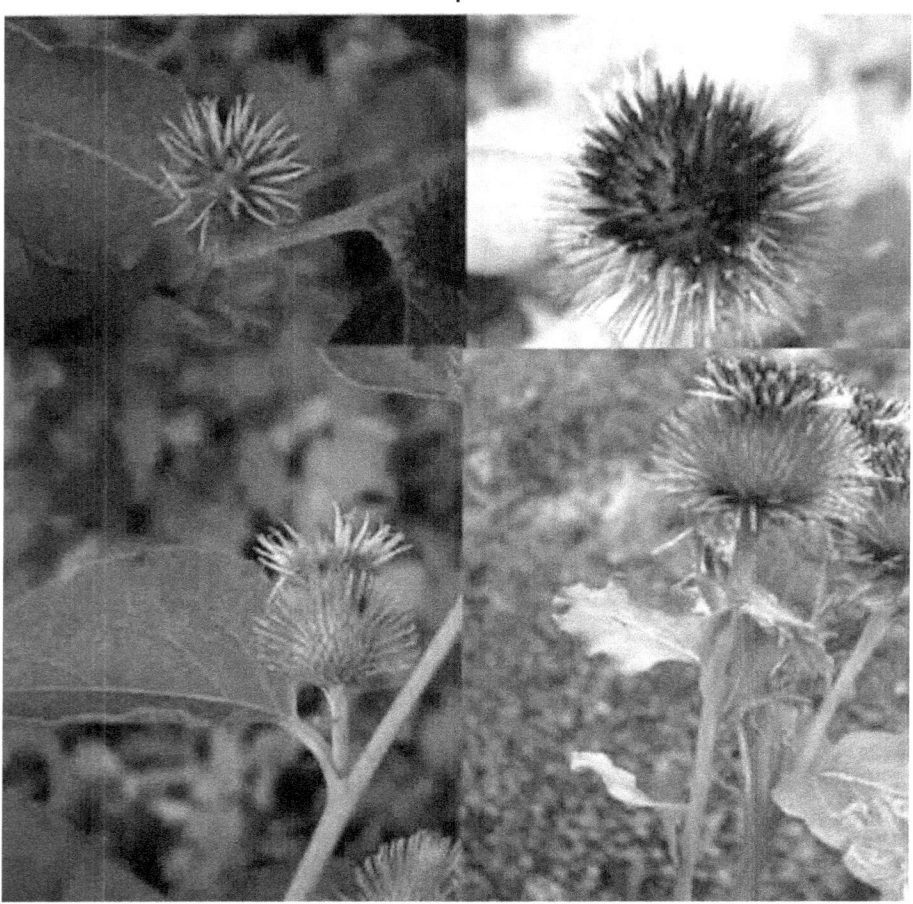

Burdock needs moist soil and sun to grow. This plant is well known as a detox in Chinese and Western holistic medicine. It is good to treat boils, rashes, herpes, bruises, acne, eczema, burns, bites, ringworm, and it requires moist soil and can grow without shade. It is well known for taking toxins out of the body that can cause infection. Please visit our website for heirloom seeds. We research the best seeds for the lowest cost.

Marigold

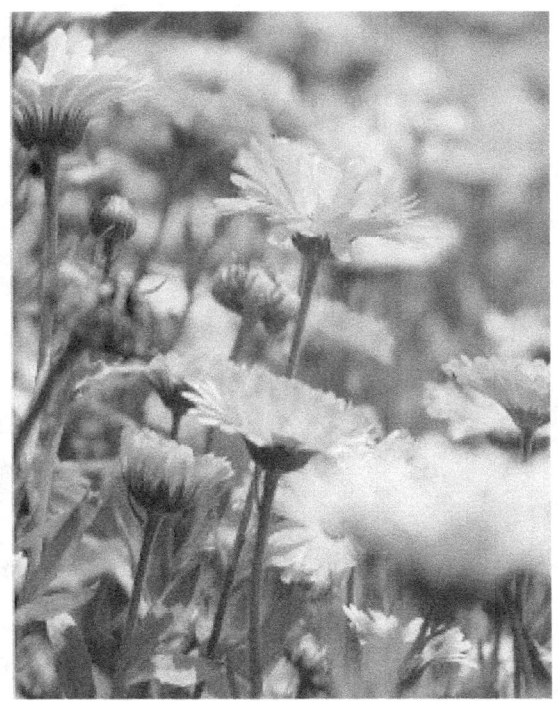

Marigold grows in any type of soil as long as it's moist. This orange little plant helps treat skin conditions and can be applied externally to bites, stings, sprains, and wounds. Internally it can treat fever or chronic infections. Make a tea and help your body have better blood circulation to prevent varicose veins. Apply externally to corns and warts and make them easily removable. Please visit our website for heirloom seeds. We research the best seeds for the lowest cost.

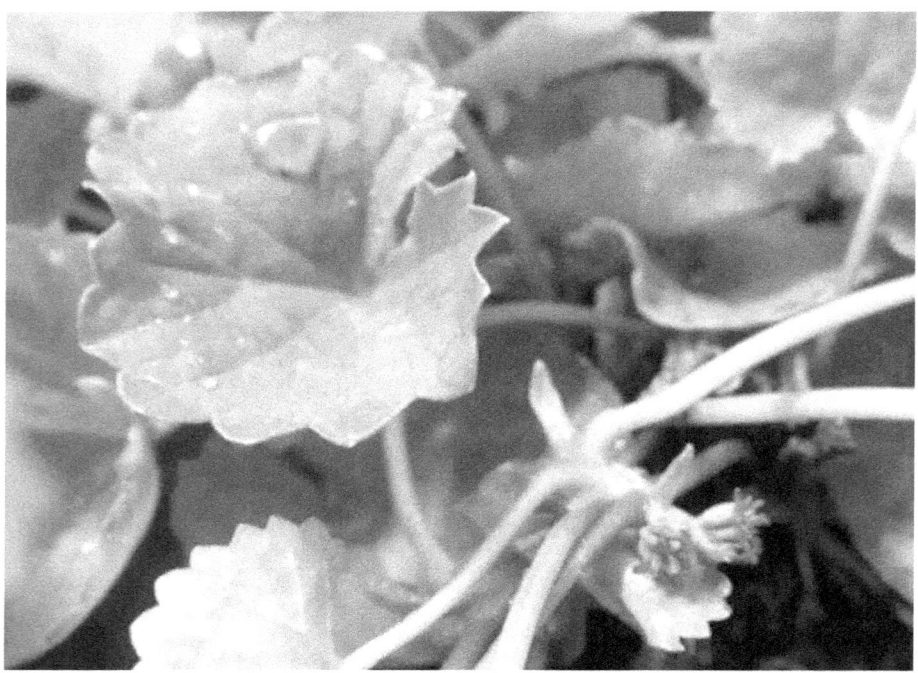

Gotu Kola heals and protects connective tissue development while stimulating healing of ulcers, skin injuries, nervous system, and open sores. It promotes healthy skin and increases attention and concentration. In ancient times, this little plant was even used to treat leprosy and maintain youthfulness.

These are just a few. Visit our website on the "Home" page for a list of easy-to-grow-in a-small-space plants that will allow you to live a long healthy life. Please visit our website for heirloom seeds. We research the best seeds for the lowest cost.

CHAPTER 9: CLOTHING

WHY WHAT YOU WEAR IS IMPORTANT CONCERNING PSORIASIS

I have wonderful thoughts every day of keeping cool. Keeping cool in hot or warm weather is an important part of happiness. Keeping cool is also important to psoriasis sufferers. Keeping cool during fall and summer is very important, when the sun is beating down, yet there is a coolness in the air; this can allow psoriasis to get worse. The reason for this is because it's harder to determine when the body is heating up. After the body heats up, it's important for the psoriasis sufferer to go inside and cool the body down. Heat makes psoriasis worse, so it's important to keep the body temperature cool at all times. That is why it is difficult to exercise during breakouts.

My journey with psoriasis was so bad that psoriasis was everywhere on my body including my face, head, arms, feet, and elbows. After many years of suffering and discovering this ancient remedy, my body became normal again. I looked in the mirror at my beautiful skin. The skin I knew I was born with but did not enjoy for many years.

I remember how detrimental heat was to my body during psoriasis breakouts. When I went to the doctor after horrible breakouts, so many times I asked, "Why does my psoriasis keep getting worse and worse in the heat?" Several doctors told me the same thing: heat makes psoriasis grow. When I got rid of my psoriasis after 35 years, it was time to go and show my beautiful skin to the world! That's when we decided to open up our company to make beautiful clothes that everybody can feel good in male or female. It is so important to be cool during the hot season and even in the winter if you live in a city or state that remains hot or warm most of the year. Our company is all about keeping cool in warm or hot weather. Something so important that hit me to the core when I had psoriasis: heat and psoriasis do not mix at all. If you overheat and have psoriasis you are doubling the discomfort and the growth of dead skin cells within a 10-minute period of time. People with psoriasis cannot exercise or be in the heat. Apparel worn during a psoriasis outbreak must be cool and loose fitting. However, it is very important to be in the sun for vitamin purposes in order to absorb vitamin C and D from your external environment. It is important that you spend short times in the sun even with psoriasis, meaning about 10 to 15 minutes a week. It is important for psoriasis sufferers to not get overheated even when in air conditioning.

We looked around the fashion industry and decided that nothing out there was really good enough to introduce my beautiful skin to the world. That is when we decided to begin a fashion line which will launch soon. Sign up for our FREE Newsletter to be the first to know at Nurse Oasis.com. We wanted to make a dress that would flatter every type of body as long as it is comfortable and fashion forward. We decided to use materials that move with the body and keep the body cool. Then we decided to make more accessories to keep the body cool. Our company will soon showcase some great fashion to keep cool with exceptional fabrics everyone will love. Our organization chooses fabrics that keep you cool, stretch with a body, and fascinating colors to make you feel good all the way around whether you're inside your home, outside gardening, or out for a night.

CONCLUSION

It is fair to say with all my research and others within our group with medical background that a majority of people with psoriasis are people that:

1. Have good character and dignity

2. Are problem solvers

3. Have empathy

4. Worry about the future and try to find solutions by prevention

5. Want to do right

6. Care about other people

7. Love with passion

8. Find relationships important

9. Care about pets

10. Love life and strive to be independent

11. A business owner or strive for new ideas in business

12. Are professional and respectful

Stress and inflammation may happen, but now there are ways to naturally prevent stress and inflammation from taking over your whole body. The best place to start is mentioned in this book. Many things may cause skin inflammation. Your body builds up toxins from stress, environment, and what you eat or drink. The body is magnificent and heals. However, as years go by, the toxins in your body accrue. The hormones released during stressful times collects proteins in the body which in turn store toxins. Eating what you grow helps, but there is still your environment. Who doesn't like to eat out, or go to an outdoor event; cry with joy or have beneficial anger?

We decided to go back, way back, when psoriasis did not exist. How did the universe help people in biblical times deal with stress? They ate natural foods. It is important to know that just eating natural foods is good, but combining natural foods is better. Also, a detox needs instructions, which we have provided in a PDF so that the meals mentioned in this book will have quicker results concerning health, well-being, and clear skin.

I want you to know after I found out about the facts written in this book, I cried for weeks, looking back at my past in amazement how I survived such a difficult childhood. After sulking in my own shell, I got up, started researching every food on a molecular level and found the most nutritious spices and foods combined that will deliver the most benefit to the body. After years of research, I finally discovered the Ancient Aztec Health and Wellness Awesome Kernel Mix and I never looked back. My life has never been the same. I hope everything mentioned in this book helps you with your psoriasis and many other ailments you may have. I wrote this book with all my heart because I wanted to help other people to get rid of psoriasis and leave it far behind. I did, and you will too. Our next project is to create a clothing line that fits our prestigious style. Stay tuned and check back at our website because we are launching soon. Better yet, sign up for our FREE Newsletter to know when we launch our clothing line and get enough vegan and non-vegan recipes to last a lifetime, plus hundreds of natural healing tips, and much more. Now, God bless you and bless your beautiful new skin!

Thank you again for purchasing this book! We hope this book was able to help you to get rid of Psoriasis for good.

The next step is to Order your Awesome Kernel Mix Today and start feeling Great Again!

Visit our website at Nurse Oasis.com for some FREE cool Natural recipes, FREE vegan and non-vegan delicious recipes to keep you healthy for a lifetime, and FREE YOGA classes for beginners!

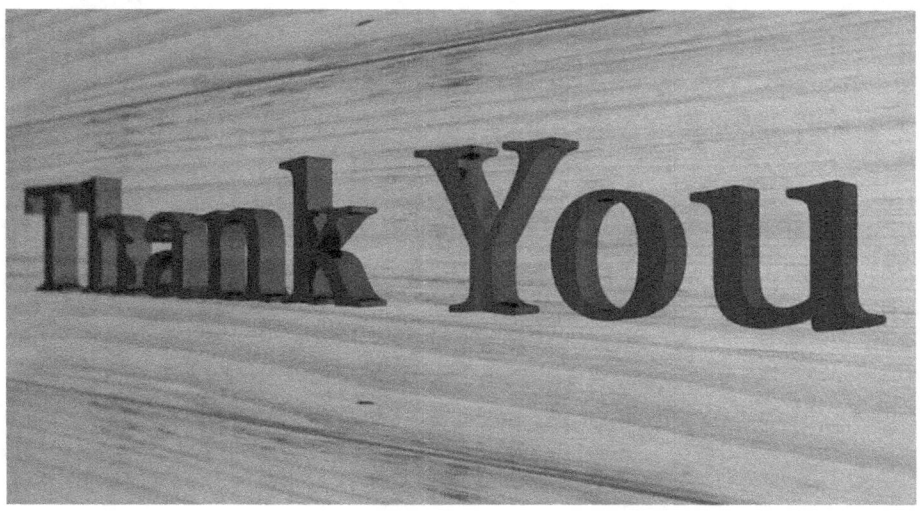

Finally, if you enjoyed this book, please leave a review on Amazon. Reviews, good or bad, allow authors to provide information to help readers. A review from you will be so greatly appreciated! Please leave a review for this book on Amazon at this link (http://amzn.to/2xdgdYG). Thank you so much!

Thank you and the Best of Health to you!

We Know you like to eat healthy! If you liked this book, check out our new "ENCHILADAS: MOST WANTED" (http://amzn.to/2xcAUDP) Book now available on Amazon! This book is a quick guide to making delicious meals every week; super simple and easy to make, and every meal is different! Great for college students and busy moms to make enchiladas QUICK! On top of that, you save tons of money eating great, healthy food at home. To Your Health!

3th TIP OF THE DAY

Having trouble Sleeping?

Try Apple Cider Vinegar and Honey as a Tea

Before bedtime, combine hot water, 2 teaspoons Apple Cider Vinegar and Honey to taste. If you put the right amount of honey, you will not even taste the Apple cider. Want to know more health benefits? Visit our website for information on how this natural, beneficial, inexpensive little mix can help you sleep and become a new person. Sleep is so important to your health and wellbeing. With this little mixture, even if you sleep 6 hours, you will wake up refreshed and rejuvenated. Be sure and do not use with medications and vitamins or at least take a week break from taking any pills before starting this little regimen.

Please leave a review for this book if it helped you in any way. Go to http://amzn.to/2xdgdYG

Do and Don'ts concerning healing from PSORIASIS

1. Do use Cream prescribed from your Doctor (Triamcinolone Acetonide Cream 01%), this will get rid of sores externally, so you can heal internally.

2. Don't take a hot bath, luke warm is better, if not cold.

3. Don't exercise or sweat until you are healed on the skin.

4. Don't wear hot clothes or clothes that make you sweat.

5. Do detox with vegetable soup, include cabbage and the Awesome Kernel Mix. Do this periodically.

6. Do find ways to relax when you are able.

7. Don't eat candy, cakes, cookies, or cokes until you are healed.

8. Do get some sun, even if it is 15 minutes a day.

9. Don't stress too much, if you consistently stress over something, remove yourself temporarily from the situation to re-coop.

10. Change your lifestyle by eating better and exercising in small increments for a longer and healthier life.

REFERENCES

1. Environmental Working Group. (2016). EWG's 2016 Dirty Dozen™ List of Pesticides on Produce: Straw berries Most Contaminated, Apples Drop to Second. <http://www.ewg.org/release/ewg-s-2016-dirty-dozen-list-pesticides-produce-strawberries-most-contaminated-apples-drop.>

2. Gilliom, Robert J., Barbash, Jack E., Crawford, Charles G., Pixie, Hamilton A., Martin, Jeffrey D., Nakagaki, Naomi, Nowell, Lisa H., Scott, Jonathan C., Stackelber, Pual E., Thelin, Gail P., Wolock David M., (2007) U.S. Geological Society. The Quality of Our Nation's Waters Pesticides in the Nation's Streams and Ground Water, 1992–2001. <https://pubs.usgs.gov/circ/2005/1291/pdf/circ1291.pdf>

3. Extoxnet.n.d., Pesticide Information Profiles. <http://extoxnet.orst.edu/pips/ghindex.html>

4. Lulla, Aaron., Barnhill, Lisa., Bitan, Gal., Magdalena, Ivanova I., Nguyen, Binh., O'Donnell, Kelley., Stahl, Mark C., Yamashiro, Chase., Frank-Gerrit Klarner, Thomas., Sagasti, Alvaro., Bronstein, Jeff M., Environmental Health Perspectives. (2016). Neurotoxicity of the Parkinson Disease-Associated Pesticide Ziram Is Synuclein-Dependent in Zebrafish Embryos. Conclusion. <https://ehp.niehs.nih.gov/ehp141/>

5. World Public Library. n.d., Pesticide in the United States. World Heritage Encyclopedia. Fungicide in the United States. WHEBN0023779733 Article No. <http://www.worldlibrary.org/articles/pesticide_use_in_the_united_states>

6. Yoquinto, Luke. (2012). The Truth About Food Additive BHA. <http://www.livescience.com/36424-food-additive-bha-butylated-hydroxyanisole.html>

7. Reuters. Science News. (2012). Study of Monsanto GM Corn Concerns Draws Skepticism.

<http://www.reuters.com/article/us-gmcrops-safety-idUSBRE88J0MS20120920>

8. Wollams, Chris. (2017). CANCER active. <http://www.canceractive.com/cancer-active-page-link.aspx?n=3148>

9. Maron, Dana F. (2015). Scientific American. Early Puberty, Causes and Effects. early Puberty. Increases in obesity appear to be the major culprit, but family stress and exposure to chemicals may also play a role. <https://www.scientificamerican.com/article/early-puberty-causes-and-effects>

10. Sprout People. n.d., The Science of Sprout Nutrition. 100% GMO Free Organic Seed Specialists Since 1993. <https://sproutpeople.org/sprouts/nutrition/science/#nutrientslegumes>

11. Dr. Axe. n.d., Marshmallow Root: The Ultimate Gut and Lung Protector. <https://draxe.com/marshmallow-root/>

12. Biddle, Wayne. (1984). Nerve Gas and Pesticides: <http://www.nytimes.com/1984/03/30/world/nerve-gases-and-pesticides-links-are-close.html>

13. Wrigley Ville Dental. (2015). Holistic Dentistry. Emotional Stress Can Cause Periodontal Disease (Gum Disease) <http://www.wrigleyvilledental.com/blog/emotional-stress-can-cause-periodontal-disease-gum-disease/>

14. Arthritis Foundation. n.d., Arthritis can Cause Different Types of Pain. <http://www.arthritis.org/living-with-arthritis/pain-management/understanding/types-of-pain.php>

15. Moyer, J.D., (2015). To Bean or Not to Bean. That is the Question. <http://www.jdmoyer.com/2011/02/15/to-bean-or-not-to-bean-that-is-//the-question-legumes-lectins-and-human-health/>